Cric Plo 3 a|a|08

EMERALD PUBLISHING

A GUIDE TO DEMENTIA CARE

Revised Edition
David Moore

Emerald Guides
www.emeraldpublishing.co.uk

Emerald Guides
Brighton BN2 4EG

ISBN: 9781847160 98 0

Printed by GN Press Ltd Essex

Cover design by Bookworks Islington

About the Author

David Moore is a trainer/ consultant. His background is in Mental Health, working with people with dementia. He has managed a number of services specifically for people with dementia including one of the first services for younger people in the UK. David has a BSc and MSc in Health Psychology and is a practising assessor and internal/ external verifier of a number of national qualifications. He currently works for West Sussex County Council, Social Services and is part of the Older Adults Mental Health Team.

Illustrated by Kirsty Moore

To my Grandad, who gave me purpose and direction.

Acknowledgements

All the staff, families and clients of, Gratwick Home Care Ltd-, Princess Marina House, Rustington Hall, St Joseph's and St Mary's Residential Homes, Hillcrest, and Tenby House.

Special thanks to:

Lisa Moulding and the staff and clients at Avon Manor – Worthing, West Sussex.

Amanda O'Hagan and the staff and clients at Avon House – Worthing, West Sussex.

Meg light – Northbrook College.

David Sheard, Peter Priednieks and Pat Kite of Dementia Care Matters Ltd, Brighton.

Anne Fretwell and Martin Lunn of Merevale House – Warwickshire

Renuka Nathan and Sister Mary and thier staff and clients at St Michaels, Nursing Home.

Darren Felgate of the Alzheimer's Society.

Jane Ralph, Andrea Linell and Kirsty Jones. West Sussex County Council, Adult Services.

Kirsty Moore, my loving wife, who has helped me during the creation of this book.

Thank you for your words and advice.

Contents

Chapter One

The Journey

I remember the first time I heard the word 'dementia'. I was ten at the time and my dad was trying to explain that my granddad had this illness. I had known for sometime that my granddad had changed; he often didn't recognise me or would confuse me with my brother or one of his sons. But it was only when he came to live with us that I realised the true affect the illness had inflicted on him. His mind had seemed to have been robbed of a lifetime of memories and skills.

Little did I know then how this experience with my granddad would shape my life? It gave me the drive to try and find out what dementia was and to understand why it had chosen someone I loved so much?

Dementia is something that affects us all. From the people who bravely live with the illness and its devastating symptoms, to those who support both the individual and their carers. Even if you don't know a person with dementia, or those who support them, at some time this growing illness will touch upon your life.

According to the Dementia UK report (2007) commissioned by the Alzheimer's society the number of people with dementia, in the UK and around the world, will dramatically increase. At the moment it is believed that there are 750,000 people with dementia in the UK. 17,500 of them are below the age of 65.

Apart from the emotional and physical consequences this will have, the economic cost is set to soar. The report currently puts the current cost, in the UK, at over 14 billion pounds a year. This growing cost is something we will all have to contribute to.

So even if you don't know a person with dementia or someone who supports them, now, the chances are that you will in the future. And of course it is possible that you may be one of those who develop dementia.

Because dementia touches upon our lives we all have a responsibility to try and understand what it is and how we can help those who are living with the journey of dementia. One of the key ways of doing this is by trying to understand what it is like to live with dementia, and hopefully this is something that this book will attain.

A journey of 'ups and downs'.

Having dementia is not a death sentence; your world is not over the day the doctor diagnoses you. The people, who I have spoken to while researching this book, have shown me this. At times it can be hell, but with the right support and understanding people with dementia and their carers can still have a life that can be full of good times.

Throughout the book there are quotes from people with dementia and their carers. These are a vital element of this book, because they are the experts, they are the ones who are living with dementia.

Quotes from people with dementia

"I am not stupid – so why do people make me feel like it?"

"It's a roller coaster… there are lots of ups and downs".

"The worst thing is worrying what will go next"?

"I am not allowed to go out…I can understand that if I go out I am a hazard".

"This isn't home….I want to go home".

"It makes me feel very tired".

"I know what's wrong. I've always known what's wrong even if they won't tell me".

"She keeps me going". (Talking about his wife).

"I look at them over there and I think that could be me next".

"I can't get it out of my head".

"You're suddenly isolated from the world if you've got dementia".

"Just because I have got this thing doesn't mean its time to give up".

"Thank god for my family".

"I don't know what the hell is the matter with me tonight….its not like it's any different from any other nights".

"Your shooed off to bed as soon as possible so they can chat and sleep. Half of me don't blame them. I mean who'd want to work with us? (A person with dementia in a care home)

"I am just plain screwed!"

Quotes from Carers

"She never speaks, but as soon as she sees a recognisable face she will laugh".

"It is hard work but it also so rewarding"

"Just the little things make a difference".

"Every day is so different, no day is the same".

"We still dance"

"Its all about holding on to what the person still has....not letting go".

"We've never talked about it in our family".

"Down in the hospital it's just like him in bed number 3. They just seem to drag them out of bed".

"She was such a lady. If she could see herself now she would commit suicide".

"Everyone seems obsessed with the paper work rather then the person".

"One so called professional said to me, 'I suppose I won't get much information out of him?' I was livid."

"I don't know what I will do once he has gone. He was...he is my life".

Furthermore this book aims to provide you with an understanding of dementia and how it affects those people who live with it.

The next chapter focuses on what dementia is and describes the different types of dementia.

The third chapter explores the symptoms of dementia and some of the possible causes.

Chapter four tries to examine the different causes of behaviour, including aggression and wandering.

The fifth chapter introduces the concept of person centred care. This type of support stresses the need to focus on the person with dementia.

Chapter six considers some of the different drug treatments that are used. The anti-dementia drugs are looked at as well as other medication such as the anti-psychotics.

Chapters seven and eight focus on some of the different support systems and therapies that may be helpful to people with dementia and their carers.

Chapter nine considers the different financial benefits that are available to people.

The final chapter contemplates the future of dementia care.

Chapter Two

Understanding Dementia

In this chapter, we will look at what dementia is and the different causes of dementia. In doing so it is hoped that a greater understanding can be gained about how a person with dementia can be affected by what is happening in their brain. Nevertheless, although it is useful to gain an understanding of the different types of dementia, it is still vital that we do not lose sight of the fact that each person with dementia is just that, a person first and foremost.

What is dementia?

The human brain is a remarkable piece of machinery that is packed full of cells that enables us to communicate with one another, feel emotions, remember past events and learn new information quicker then any computer. Despite the brain's brilliance, like any part of our body, there are times when it can be affected by disease.

There are a number of different diseases that can cause a person's brain cells, and their connections to one another, to become damaged and stop working. This can result in a person experiencing a serious decline in their ability to remember, communicate with others, think clearly and undertake every day activities. This decline in mental abilities is referred to as dementia.

In everyone's brain...... ......there are billions of cells.

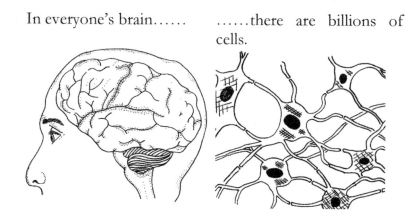

But in dementia the cells, ...are slowly destroyed.
....

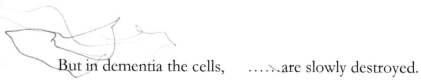

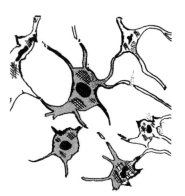

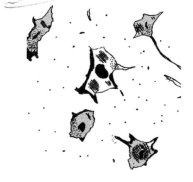

Currently there is no cure for the majority of the causes of dementia, although there are treatments that can help with some of the symptoms. (This is looked at in chapter six). However some causes of dementia can potentially be treated, such as hypothyroidism (under active thyroid gland), brain tumours and vitamin deficiency. Unfortunately it is not until a post mortem is performed and the brain is studied under the microscope, that a diagnosis can be given for definite.

MYTHS ABOUT DEMENTIA – OLD AGE CAUSES DEMENTIA

It was once believed that dementia was a normal part of getting old. This is now known not to be true because dementia can affect people at any age, including young children. (A very rare genetic children's condition called Neiman's Pick disease type c can cause dementia).
However age is a risk factor. In other words the older you are the more likely you are to develop dementia.

An umbrella term.

Dementia is a serious condition, just like heart disease or cancer. As with cancer, there are lots of different types or causes of dementia. Consequently dementia is often referred to as an umbrella term i.e. a word that covers a number of different conditions that cause a person to experience a similar set of symptoms.

The following picture shows some of the different conditions that can come under the umbrella of dementia.

Dementia

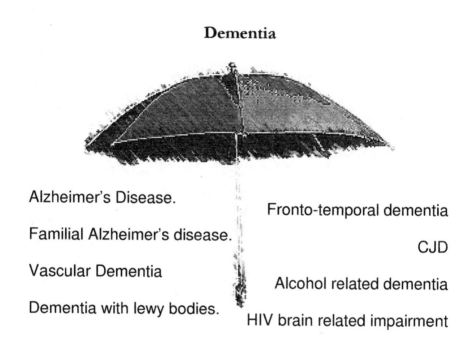

Alzheimer's Disease.

Fronto-temporal dementia

Familial Alzheimer's disease.

CJD

Vascular Dementia

Alcohol related dementia

Dementia with lewy bodies.

HIV brain related impairment

Dementia is not uncommon. According to the Alzheimer's Society there are approximately 800,000 people with dementia in the UK. Alzheimer's disease accounts for almost half of that figure as demonstrated in the following table.

See Table One Overleaf.

Table One. Types and Numbers

Type of dementia	Approx number of people with type of dementia	What causes brain damage
Alzheimer's disease	450,000	A person's brain cells are attacked by abnormalities called plaques and tangles. There is also a reduction of a chemical in the brain cells.
Vascular dementia	200,000	The brain cells are destroyed by diseased blood vessels or by being deprived of oxygen. (It is possible to have both vascular dementia and Alzheimer's disease).
Dementia with Lewy bodies	100,000	The brain is attacked by a gradual build up of protein deposits – known as Lewy bodies.
Fronto-temporal dementia.	11,000	Cells become swollen

The symptoms of the different types of dementia will be looked at in chapter 3 but now we will go on to look at these different types in more detail.

Alzheimer's disease

The symptoms of Alzheimer's disease were first described by a German doctor back in 1902. The doctor's name was Alois Alzheimer's and his patient was a woman known only as Auguste D. Before her death, Auguste had shown a number of symptoms, we now associate with Alzheimer's disease.

After Auguste's death Dr Alzheimer's performed an examination of her brain to try and understand the possible causes of these symptoms. He found that a number of cells in Auguste's brain had died or were seriously damaged. He discovered that this damage was caused by deposits of protein known as **amyloid plaques** and **tau tangles.**

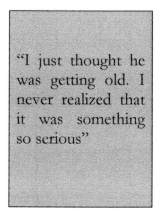

"I just thought he was getting old. I never realized that it was something so serious"

These deadly proteins gradually grow in number and wage a war against the person with Alzheimer's brain cells and their connections to one another. Tau protein attacks the cells from inside, causing tangles to form. This causes the cells to swell up like a balloon, until they explode and die. Amyloid protein causes plaques to form outside of the cell. These plaques then grow like ivy slowly suffocating the cell.

Working together, these plaques and tangles lead to certain areas of a person's brain being severely damaged and in some cases destroyed altogether. This damage firstly occurs in the memory part of the brain, hence the first symptom of short-term memory loss. Then the plaques and tangles spread to other parts of the brain resulting in the other symptoms of Alzheimer's, including personality changes, difficulties with walking and loss of mental abilities such as reading and writing.

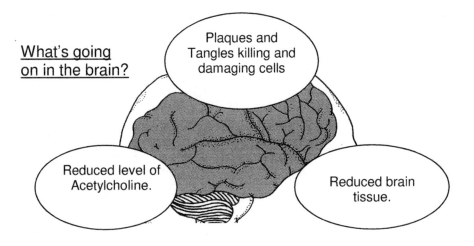

What's going on in the brain?

Plaques and Tangles killing and damaging cells

Reduced level of Acetylcholine.

Reduced brain tissue.

The spread of plaques and tangles usually happens over along period of time, and at first people may put their symptoms down to getting old or stress. It is only later on that people usually recognise these signs are something more serious then stress.

Further research has shown that people with Alzheimer's face another challenge. This is because the brain cells have a reduced level of a chemical called Acetylcholine. Without this chemical the brain cells find it a lot harder to communicate with one another.

Vascular Dementia

Vascular dementia is an umbrella term in itself used to describe a number of illnesses that affects the bodies' vascular system which results in a poor blood supply to the brain. Our brain needs this supply of blood to provide it with oxygen and nutrients. The vascular system does this by sending blood vessels to the brain via a network of arteries. A bit like lots of canal boats (the blood vessels) carrying oxygen on a group of different canals (the arteries).

For the blood vessels to get to the brain they need an unobstructed path and a healthy heart to pump them there. Consequently heart disease, high blood pressure or blockages to the arteries can affect the blood supply and so cause cells in the brain to starve to death leading to vascular dementia

The commonest cause of vascular dementia is a stroke. A stroke happens when a blockage in an artery stops the blood getting to the brain or when the artery itself becomes damaged. This causes the brain cells to die or become damaged and causes the symptoms of dementia. Not everyone who has a stroke will develop dementia - this often depends on the part of the brain that is damaged.

If damage occurs to the brain as a result of lots of little strokes then this is called **Multi-infarct dementia**. These repeated strokes cause a build up of damage in a person's brain. The affect these strokes have on a person's abilities depend on how much damage occurs to the brain a result of each stroke

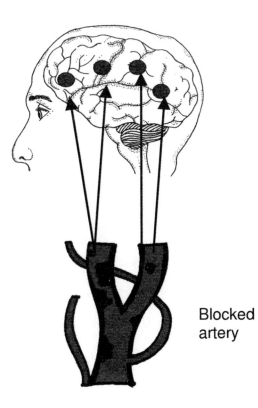

Blocked
artery

****

If dementia occurs as the result of one big stroke it is known as **Single-infarct dementia.** This will then affect one distinct area of the brain.

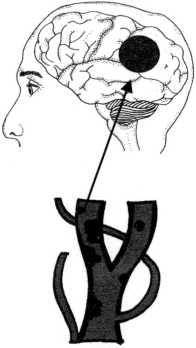

****

Also the blood vessels themselves can be diseased and damaged, which stops them from doing their job properly. This happens as a result of the arteries becoming narrow and hard.

"After the stroke he became very low. He wouldn't even talk to his best friend who he had known for years"

This hardening can be caused by smoking, age, high blood pressure and cholesterol. As the arteries become narrower less blood gets to the brain causing damage. When this happens it is known as Binswanger's disease or subcortical dementia. Often doctors will try to slow down the narrowing of the arteries and so slow down the progression of Binswanger's disease. This can be done by following a healthy life style and medication.

Dementia with Lewy Bodies

Dementia with lewy bodies is referred to by many other names including lewy body disease, lewy body dementia and diffuse lewy body disease.

This type of dementia is caused by an abnormal build up of protein, known as lewy bodies, which develops inside of and destroys brain cells. They are named after the doctor who first discovered the deposits while researching Parkinson's disease, Dr Friedrich Heinrich Lewy, who was a colleague of Alois Alzheimer's.

In Parkinson's disease lewy bodies are usually found in the brain stem where they attack a chemical called dopamine. This causes symptoms of Parkinson's disease such as rigidity, stiffness and tremors. However Dr Lewy found that in some cases these lewy bodies spread to other parts of the brain, which caused the symptoms of dementia. Hence the name dementia with lewy bodies.

The Fronto-temporal dementias.

Fronto-temporal dementia relates to a number of different dementias that include Pick's disease, semantic dementia, frontal lobe degeneration and primary progressive aphasia.

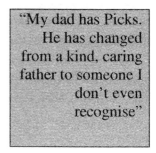

"My dad has Picks. He has changed from a kind, caring father to someone I don't even recognise"

These types of dementia affect specific parts of the brain called the frontal and the temporal lobes. As a result, in the early experience of the illnesses, a person's personality and behaviour will be affected rather then their memory. This can change later on in the illness.

Picks disease was identified by a doctor, called Arnold Pick. He discovered that in the brains of people with this type of dementia that their cells were unusual in shape and swollen. He called these cells Pick cells. Also Dr Pick identified a build up of protein, which he called Pick bodies. As in the plaques and tangles, seen in Alzheimer's disease, these Pick bodies & Pick cells work together to cause the death of a person's cells located in the front part of the brain.

People with **semantic dementia** often have problems using or understanding the meaning of words. For example a person could be shown a picture of a clock and they would not be able to tell you what it was. Furthermore they would have difficulty in telling you information about what the clock was used for, i.e. you used it to tell the time. This type of dementia generally affects the temporal lobe of the brain. Some elements of speech are located in the frontal lobe. Damage to localized areas of this lobe can cause a person to develop **Primary Progressive Aphasia.** In other words a person's ability to use speech will gradually become worse. It is not until later on in the illness that a person will have problems with their memory and personality.

Familial Fronto- temporal dementia is thought to be genetic. Research has indicated that there may be a problem with some of the genes on chromosomes 3 and 17.

Creutzfeldt-Jakob Disease (CJD)

This is another group of illness that is thought to be caused by a PRION attacking a person's brain cells. A prion is an infectious item made only of protein. Too much of the wrong protein causes serious damage to the brain.

Because a prion is infectious this means it can be spread in different ways. It has been suggested that it could be passed through infected meat. This is known as New Variant CJD and it is thought to be connected to BSE ('mad cow disease'). This type of dementia causes a person to decline very quickly. Often the person will die as a result of CJD in a very short amount of time, usually about 1 year.

It is also possible for the prion to be passed through genes. This type of CJD is called Familial CJD. In families where CJD is present genetic counseling can often be offered.

Case example: Jo

Jo was 14 when her mother, Sarah, was diagnosed with familial CJD. After a few years of trying to look after her at home Jo's father decided to move Sarah into a small home for younger people with dementia.

Jo had been offered genetic counseling through the home but she had refused. However when Jo fell pregnant she became concerned that she would pass the illness onto her unborn child. Consequently Jo decided to undertake the counseling to try and help to decide whether to keep the baby. Eventually Jo decided to have a termination because she felt that the risk was too high.

Although CJD has been heavily mentioned in the media it is still very rare and only affects one person in a million in the UK each year.

Alcohol related dementia.

Brain cells can become damaged as a result of serious alcohol abuse. This damage can cause the person to have a number of problems including with memory and keeping their balance. It is still not known for definite if it is the alcohol that damages the brain cells directly or if it is because of the lack of thiamine (vitamin B1), which is destroyed by alcohol.

Not everyone who drinks large amounts of alcohol will develop alcohol related dementia, but it does increase the risk of this dementia developing.

> "My uncle had always had a drink problem, but recently he has even had trouble walking and remembering the simplest things"

In the early stages of alcohol related dementia it has been suggested that it may be possible to reduce further damage to the person's brain by encouraging the person to stop drinking, to improve their diet and to take thiamine supplements.

HIV brain related impairment.

HIV brain related impairment (also known as **AIDS dementia complex** or **HIV associated dementia)** is only found in people with HIV. The HIV virus attacks the brain cells causing the cells to die. This is a very rare type of dementia and research is ongoing.

Dementia in Huntington's disease.

Huntington's is an inherited disease that causes damage to the nervous system and certain areas of the brain. This is caused by a faulty gene that can be passed from a person with Huntington's disease to their child. Some people with Huntington's can develop dementia and consequently have problems with their memory and learning new information.

Dementia Pugilistica

There is a possible link between head injuries and a particular type of dementia known as Dementia Pugilistica or as 'boxer's dementia'. It has received this name because it is commonly found in individuals who have participated in sports that involve continual blows to the head, such as boxing.

> **QUESTION.** IS PARKINSON'S DISEASE A TYPE OF DEMENTIA?
>
> Parkinson's disease is not a type of dementia. People with Parkinson's do not usually have problems with their short-term memory. Nevertheless a small percentage of people with Parkinson's can go on to develop dementia.
>
> Consequently a person will not only have difficulty with their movement but they will also have problems with their mental abilities.

This second chapter has looked at some of the different types of dementia. In the next chapter we will go onto look at the different causes and symptoms of these types.

34

Chapter Three

Causes and Symptoms

This third chapter aims to look at some symptoms of dementia and some symptoms that are specific to the different types of dementia. Some of the possible causes of dementia will be examined.

No two people are the same.

There are a number of different symptoms that the majority of the forms of dementia have in common. Despite this, no two people will experience the symptoms of dementia in the same way. This is because everyone with dementia is so different to begin with. Many factors will play a part in the person's experience of dementia including:

- The form of dementia
- The person's experiences and personality
- How the person is treated by others such as their family.
- If the person has any other illnesses.
- The support they receive- such as medical treatment.

Despite the differences the majority of the dementia's are progressive. This means that it will become harder over time for a person with dementia as their brain becomes more damaged. Nevertheless the one thing a person with dementia will always have is their ability to feel a wide range of feelings and emotions.

Symptoms of dementia.

Some of the general signs and symptoms of dementia include:

- **Memory Problems**.

Memory loss can be one of the fundamental symptoms of dementia, in particular of Alzheimer's disease. Early on a person with dementia may only experience slight problems with their memory such as forgetting telephone numbers or where they have put things, such as their car keys.

As dementia progresses noticeable memory problems occur that are severe enough to affect a person's daily life. The person may not remember that they have eaten or they may struggle to undertake tasks such as driving and preparing a meal. A person may remember parts of an ability such as cooking a meal, but not the whole sequence from start to finish. For example a person may remember to switch the oven on but then forget to put anything in the oven.

"I knew something was seriously wrong when he walked home from the supermarket. This would have been fine but he had driven there"

Later on the memory loss may become even more distressing for the person and their family as they struggle to remember what their friends and relatives look like.

Nevertheless forgetting things occasionally does not mean that a person has dementia; memory loss is something that happens to us all. We need to do this to get rid of information that is not useful to us.

However if memory loss is frequent, I.e. if a person continually looses their keys, or regularly asks similar questions over a period of time then it is certainly worth speaking to general practitioner. Even this type of forgetting is not necessarily a confirmation that the person has dementia. Numerous factors can cause such memory loss, including other illnesses and certain forms of medication.

A trip down Memory Lane.

Although, in dementia, a person's ability to remember recent information is impaired, not all forms of memory are as badly affected. For instance emotional memory remains in tact. This refers to the ability to remember feelings and emotions. Consequently a person may forget recent events because of their short term memory loss but they will not forget how the event made them feel e.g., angry, happy, sad etc. This demonstrates why it is still important to involve a person with dementia with others and in activities. Even if they forget the conversation or the activity they will not forget how it made them feel – hopefully good.

Also many people with dementia will have good long-term memory. It may seem strange that a person with dementia may not remember what happened recently but they can still recall facts and information from years ago.

To help understand why this is it is worth thinking of memories as a road or a lane. As we grow we learn from our experiences and these are stored as memories to help us on our journey. Memories keep getting added and the lane keeps getting longer.

At the end of the lane recent memories are stored, but the further we go back down the lane the older the memories are. In the brain recent memories are kept on the surface and old memories are stored deep in the brain.

As dementia attacks the surface of a person's brain it sweeps away the recent memories. The dementia has to brush away all of the recent memories before it can get to the long-term memories. Consequently the memories of a person's past are still there and are still protected.

Dementia –
Sweeping away the
recent memories

Short term
Memories-
surface of the
brain

Long-term memories
– Deep in the brain

****

It can be frustrating when a person with dementia repeats himself or herself or asks a question over and over. Although you might tell the person the answer they may soon forget what you have said because the information has been swept away.

• Losing things regularly

All of us lose things, possible even on a daily basis. However for people with dementia this may happen frequently during the day because of poor short-term memory. People may forget that they have moved an item and so accuse others of taking their possessions. This can lead to feelings of insecurity and paranoia.

• Judgment.

A person with dementia can have problems with making decisions and judgments. This can range from their ability to make judgments about what to wear to being able to judge if they are safe to undertake potentially risky activities such as driving.

If a person's judgment is affected then they can make a number of poor decisions, such as driving the wrong way down the motorway, wearing summer clothes in winter or giving money to strangers.

- **Disorientation.**

This refers to person's uncertainness about their surroundings. A person may become lost in familiar surroundings because of their failing short term memory. Similarly a person may become confused about the time of day, the month or the year.

> "I could tell how hard he was trying to tell me from the look on his face"

Many people with dementia, who are in familiar surroundings, can still function well. For instance if a person has lived in the same house for many years it is very likely that they will be able to remain at home for a long time. This is because they are in a familiar environment following familiar routines. However the person will still need support especially when faced with new challenges.

- **Communication difficulties.**

Early on a person with dementia may struggle with finding the right words or they may repeat themselves. For example a person may have difficulty in naming an object such as a cup or a pair of trousers. Later on a person may lose the ability to talk and to understand what is being said to them. This is known as aphasia or dysphasia.

- **Apraixa**

This refers to when a person's brain does not tell their body how to carry out a task. For instance a person knows what they want to do, e.g. have a cup of tea, but they can't recall what steps need

40

to be taken to make a cup of tea. Apraxia can result in a person having a number of problems such as putting their clothes on in the wrong order or having difficulty with cooking a meal.

Despite a number of symptoms being shared there are some distinct differences, which will now be looked at.

Symptoms of Alzheimer's disease

The first symptom of Alzheimer's is short-term memory loss. People with Alzheimer's disease can also experience problems with:

- Recognising familiar voices or the meaning of tones of voice, like knowing when a person is angry or happy.
- Writing and, in some cases, reading, or carrying out simple arithmetical tasks.
- Personality changes. For example if the person was quiet they may become very loud and outgoing.

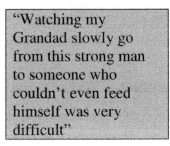

"Watching my Grandad slowly go from this strong man to someone who couldn't even feed himself was very difficult"

As the disease advances individuals may become more frustrated and frightened especially when faced with difficulties with eating or controlling their bladder and/ or bowel.

The progression of Alzheimer's disease will be different for each person.

41

Symptoms of Vascular dementia

The symptoms of vascular dementia often depend on which area of the brain has been affected and how badly damaged this area is.

In the early stages of vascular dementia a person may not experience the same memory difficulties as in Alzheimer's disease and so have a greater awareness of the difficulties they are experiencing. Such difficulties can include:

- Problems with walking,
- Seizures and tremors.
- Problems with communication such as slurred speech or repetitiveness.

Case study: Kim

Kim had become more worried about her dad, Mike, since the death of her mother two years ago. She knew he was having problems with his memory but she had put it down to his age. Kim didn't see her dad as often as she would have liked because he lived over 200 miles away in Sussex. However when he rang her for the fifth time that month to ask her where her mother was she realized that there was something seriously wrong.

> "I hate what is happening to me. I hate it…I hate it!"

As a result of this awareness vascular dementia is often accompanied by depression. Having depression can make a person's concentration, memory and attention worse.

However, with the right help and treatment many people can recover from depression. A person who experiences vascular dementia as a result of a number of strokes may find that their symptoms happen in a step process. In other words the person loses ability after a stroke then they are fine until another stroke occurs and consequently another ability is lost.

Person has a stroke and experiences a decline in abilities.

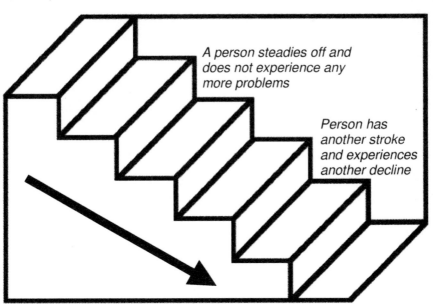

A person steadies off and does not experience any more problems

Person has another stroke and experiences another decline

Symptoms in dementia with Lewy bodies.

People with dementia with lewy bodies can have similar symptoms to both Alzheimer's disease, memory problems, and Parkinson's disease, problems with movement. However dementia with lewy bodies also has other symptoms including:

• A roller coaster of impairment.

A person with dementia with lewy bodies can experience a roller coaster of ups and downs through out the day. There may be times when a person can remember and be aware of their surroundings but this may change later on in the day.

• Hallucinations.

Many people with this type of dementia experience hallucinations, seeing things that are not there. Although hallucinations can occur in other types of dementia it is more common in dementia with lewy bodies.

> "She kept saying that there were spiders in her room. She wouldn't sleep in there no matter how many times I told her there weren't any. She ended up sleeping in the front room on the settee"

Some people may be aware that they are hallucinations where as others may become very distressed by them because they seem so real.

• Problems with sleep.

Some people with dementia with lewy bodies can stay awake for long periods of time. This can be very stressful both for the person and their carer.

Symptoms of Fronto-temporal dementia

Because these types of dementia affect the front part of the brain, the symptoms seen are related to the function of these areas. The front part of our brain tells us what behaviour is socially acceptable and what is not. Damage to this part of the brain may result in a person not acting 'appropriately'. For example they may take their clothes off in front of others, talk to complete to strangers about private matters, become sexually suggestive or may take other peoples property without seeking their permission. Often though a person may not realise their behaviour is offending others or is seen as inappropriate. Also a person with fronto-temporal dementia may:

- Experience a severe change in personality.
- Start to follow obsessive routines, such as over eating, over spending or constant cleaning.

Now some of the symptoms have been discussed the potential causes of dementia will be explored.

Causes of Dementia

For the majority of the forms of dementias we still do not know the cause, although there have been a numerous suggestions. It is suspected that dementia may be caused by a combination of factors, such as genetics and social factors. Furthermore there may be factors that increase a person's risk of developing dementia; such as old age or the type of life style we lead.

Genetics.

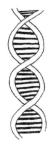

Our DNA (the building blocks of who we are) is passed down to us from our parents in the form of **GENES**. Genes carry information about a person's development from parents to children. Sometimes genes carry information that is not always wanted such as an illness like dementia

It is thought that genetics may play a strong part in a number of cases of people with dementia. Research has looked at a number of chromosome's including numbers 21, 19, 14, and 10.

However there are many cases of dementia where no one else in the family has had dementia. This means that there must be other reasons why people develop dementia other than just genetics.

QUESTION. DO GENETICS CAUSE ALZHEIMER'S?

Familial Alzheimer's disease (FAD) is a type of Alzheimer's disease where the cause seems to be genetic. However this type of Alzheimer's disease only accounts for about 5 – 10% of total cases. This suggests that genetics is only a cause of Alzheimer's disease in a small number of cases.

Social Factors.

Recently research has focused on the influence a person's lifestyle has on the chances of developing dementia. It is already known that an unhealthy life style increases the risk of developing heart disease, diabetes or of having a stroke and therefore vascular dementia. It is also known that severe alcohol abuse can cause alcohol related dementia. However the relationship between life style and the other types of dementia is still not clear.

Different food items have been looked at including oily fish, garlic and caffeine, to see if eating these can reduce the risk of developing dementia. However research is still ongoing.

Another area that has been researched is the possible link between mobiles and dementia. Back in 2003 Swedish researchers claimed that mobiles caused Alzheimer's disease.

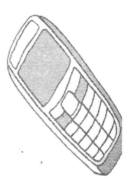

Although there may be concern about the use of mobiles it is worth knowing that many studies were undertaken on rats in a laboratory situation and so it may be difficult to apply the results to human beings.

Nevertheless it may possible that regular use of mobiles over a long period of time may cause Alzheimer's.

Other potential causes of dementia that have been looked at include:

- **Pollution.**
- **Snoring.** Leeds University School of medicine recently suggested that heavy snoring could cause dementia due to lack of oxygen.

47

- **Whiplash.** Researchers at the University of Pennsylvania have claimed that whiplash may cause Alzheimer's.
- **Problems with the immune system.** Some scientists think that Dementia may be similar to diseases of the autoimmune system such as Multiple Sclerosis. It is possible that as the brain ages the immune system attacks the brain cells because it believes they are intruders. However research into this theory is still inconclusive.
- **Repeated blows to the head**

So it seems that there are many ideas about what can cause dementia but still very little conclusive evidence to tell us why some people get dementia and others do not.

MYTHS ABOUT DEMENTIA
Aluminum causes dementia?

This was once thought to be true because in some people with dementia's brain, this metal was found. However further research has indicated that it is very unlikely that Aluminium causes dementia.

The next chapter will look as some of the behaviors shown by people with dementia.

Chapter Four

Understanding Behaviour

One of the hardest challenges faced in caring for people with dementia is trying to cope with and understand a person's change in behaviour. Often families describe caring for someone who shows difficult behaviour as a major challenge and this can put a great deal of strain on the relationship. This chapter aims to try and understand the reasons for such behaviour and focuses on the need to understand rather then manage or control the behaviour.

Difficult behaviour

The terms challenging and difficult behaviour have been used to describe actions shown by people with dementia that are particularly difficult to cope with or to understand. These terms often refer to behaviour such as aggression and wandering.

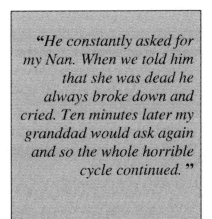

"He constantly asked for my Nan. When we told him that she was dead he always broke down and cried. Ten minutes later my granddad would ask again and so the whole horrible cycle continued."

Aggression

Probably the behaviour carers find most difficult to handle is aggression; this is often because the consequences of an aggressive act can have a long lasting affect on a carer both physically and emotionally.

These affects can be magnified if the person with dementia has never showed aggression before the illness.

Aggression can affect the person with dementia also. If a person remembers being aggressive they may struggle to understand why they have acted this way, especially if it is a change in their personality. Even if a person can't remember they may be only too aware of the fall out after the incident.

> *"He never lost his temper, never! Now it is like waiting for a ticking time bomb to go off."*

Case study: Mr. Hatton

Mr. Hatton was a seventy two year old man who had Alzheimer's disease. His memory and verbal skills had been severely affected. Before his illness Mr. Hatton had never been aggressive, however over the last six months this had changed. His aggression was usually towards his wife, Rebecca.

Rebecca was exhausted and was struggling to cope. Consequently Rebecca contacted her husbands GP who referred her husband to a psychiatrist. Consequently Mr. Hatton was admitted him to a local mental health unit for assessment. While in hospital he was not aggressive towards the staff or other patients.

Mr. Hatton returned home with extra support from a community mental health nurse. However he became aggressive again towards his wife. After spending time with Mr. Hatton the nurse discovered that he believed that Rebecca was a stranger in his home. Rebecca tried to explain that she was his wife but this only made him angrier. As a result the Nurse suggested that Mr. Hatton should go to a local day centre to give Rebecca a break. She also suggested a course that Rebecca could go to try and defuse her husband's anger.

Although the aggression still occurred the course had given Rebecca more confidence in identifying what caused her husband's behaviour.

Aggression can happen for many reasons, some may be more obvious then others. If a person is aggressive it is important to try not to make the situation worse. All of us are wound up by certain actions of others, especially when we're feeling angry or upset. For example being stared at, shouted at or being told to calm down or to be reasonable usually only adds fuel to the fire.

However the key difference between people without dementia and those with dementia is that the aggression cannot be controlled in the same way. This is because their brain is damaged. This does not stop the aggression being any less worrying or scary but it does help us consider how we should react to aggression. Punishing or scolding a person for being aggressive may not be helpful because they will forget both the incident of aggression and the resulting punishment. However they may not forget the feelings the punishment created in them, possibly anger. This anger then may build through out the day until it is again expressed through aggression.

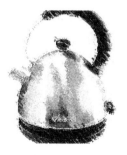

Often people with dementia do not have the opportunity to express anger. Usually the first signs of aggression are met with attempts at calming the person. However aggression can be like steam in a kettle. If it does not have opportunity to be released in small controlled amounts then it will boil over.

A person with dementia can be helped to release their anger in a controlled way, through things such as exercise. This will not help everyone but may be useful for some.

Repetitiveness

Repetitiveness refers to when a person with dementia repeats a word, phrase or action.

Though to a carer this may feel like a deliberate act, the person with dementia is often unaware of their action and do not understand the consequences that arise.

People with dementia have genuinely forgotten either asking the question or the answer they received, and if greeted with an angry response, may see this as an unreasonable reaction to a question. People try and cope with this in different ways. Some people have a written answer for the person with dementia to read, other people try diverting the person's attention on to something else.

Inappropriate behaviour

Some people with dementia may loose their inhibitions and so find it difficult to judge what is socially acceptable or tactful. For instance a person with dementia who starts to undress in a doctor's waiting room or tries to kiss a complete stranger or tells rude jokes at church may be greeted with shock and embarrassment.

Wandering or walking?

Carers often find a person's wandering particularly distressing especially if the person with dementia wanders away from home at night. In such cases a carer may believe the only option is lock the doors and hide the keys to prevent a person from roaming the streets at night.

Many care homes have a locked door policy however other establishments have invested in technology that alerts staff if a person with dementia leaves the environment by calling staff pagers or sounding an alarm.

Because many people will remain physically able, preventing walking around or access to the outside world during the day may lead to a person becoming frustrated and possibly aggressive. Therefore many care homes give consideration to giving opportunity for activities outside the home. Also risk assessments are undertaken. This is done to identify potential hazards and allow steps to be taken to reduce the risk of someone being harmed by such hazards.

Attachment behaviours.

According to the psychologist Bowlby, the need for attachment to others is just as important to human development as vitamins. We all have a need for attachment and just because an individual develops dementia does not mean that this need suddenly disappears. In fact having dementia may increase this need for security and comfort.

This need may lead to a person with dementia constantly following a particular individual, which can be a great source of distress for that person. Or a person may regularly ask for another individual such as their mother or father.

Question. Is Challenging behaviour a useful term to use?

Some people have argued that the term 'challenging or difficult behaviour' creates a number of issues. Including:

1   It conjures up a very negative view of people with dementia and makes us think that behaviours are something specific to people with dementia. All of us show behaviours that can challenge others, this is not exclusive to people with dementia.

2   It does not consider other types of behaviour, which may not be challenging for carers. For example someone sitting in the corner quietly may be trying to express a need, but this is often ignored because the person is not being 'difficult'.

> 3 The behaviour may not be challenging to everyone. For example one member of staff may find a person who regularly walks around challenging because they are worried that the person could fall. However another member of staff may think it is a good idea because the person is getting regular exercise.

Reasons For Behaviour.

It was originally presumed that behaviours such as 'wandering' were symptoms of dementia. It is now understood that people are doing this because they are relying on their behaviour as a form of communication, as it may be the only language they have left to tell others about a need or feeling.

Behaviour is how a person with dementia attempts to communicate with us, so it is important that we try to understand what they are telling us. The first step in this understanding, is to realise there is a reason behind the behaviour. The person is not just being awkward – although it may feel like this at times.

One possible reason behind a person's behaviour is due to the changes that have occurred in the brain. Damage to a person's brain prevents it from working, as it should, which can lead to a number of unusual behaviours occurring.

The Frontal Lobe: The Social Controller.

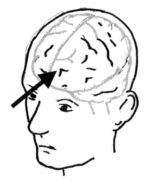

Damage to the front part of the brain, known as the frontal lobe, can cause a person to act in a way that is not socially or culturally acceptable. For instance a person who never swore before the illness may start to use colourful language or become rude or abusive.

A person's sexual behaviour may become more explicit or a person's understanding of social eating may alter. A person may undress in front of others, without realising that it is 'socially inappropriate' to do so in this situation.

FACT
A Portuguese doctor, called Egas Moniz, developed a technique of removing parts of the frontal lobe known as Frontal lobotomy. It was discovered that the patients had radical changes in personality, leading to unusual behaviour. This demonstrated the frontal lobes role in personality.

When a person shows such behaviour, the first instinct may be to tell the person off or to stop it. However this may not be helpful. This is because damage to their short term memory will prevent the person from learning. Inevitably a person may soon forget what has been said and only remember the feelings they are left with, such as embarrassment or anger.

Furthermore, highlighting to the person that they have behaved in this way will possibly heighten their feeling of embarrassment.

It is worth trying to consider why has the person behaved in this way in the first place. For example has the person undressed because:

- They are too hot?
- They are uncomfortable in the clothes they are wearing?
- They need the toilet?
- They do not realise that they are surrounded by other people.

All of this unsociable behaviour can be because the frontal lobe is not doing its job correctly; it is unable to judge how to act in certain situations.

Also damage to the front part of the brain can mean that a person could have problems with

- Making decisions, such as what to wear, what time to catch a bus, what to do in an emergency etc.
- Planning how to get somewhere, how to cook a meal or what do to keep busy.
- Solving problems such as deciding how to over come obstacles, who to call if in trouble.

The Temporal Lobe

Another part of the brain that can be affected in dementia is the temporal lobe. This is found beneath the frontal and parietal lobe and is involved in understanding and processing sound.

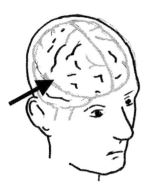

The temporal lobe also contains a part of the brain known as the hippocampus. This small area of the brain is involved both in memory and spatial navigation, being able to get us around without becoming lost.

In Alzheimer's disease it is the hippocampus that is affected first which explains the early symptoms of disorientation and memory loss.

If this part of the brain is damaged then you might see a person with dementia showing a number of behaviours due to their memory problems, such as repeating themselves or becoming lost.

The Parietal Lobe

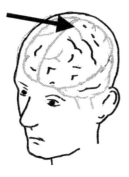

This area is found just above the temporal and occipital lobes. This part of the brain is mainly involved with making sense of sensory information, such as sound, touch and taste. Damage to this area may explain why some people with dementia repeat themselves – because they can not make sense of the answers they are given.

The parietal lobe also helps us to use and understand language. If this part of the brain becomes damaged, a person can have major problems with language. This can cause great frustration for people with dementia.

The Occipital Lobe.

This part of the brain is involved in helping us make sense of what we see around us. If this part of the brain becomes damaged then a person could have problems understanding what they are seeing. For example a person may :

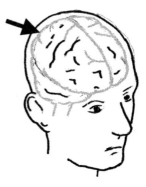

- Misinterpret a floral pattern in a carpet as an animal or a face.
- Think that black squares on the floor are holes and so refuse to walk on the floor.

59

- Not see the toilet because the white toilet seat, the white toilet and the white floor all blend into one.
- Take a large step over a floor joining because they think it is a step. Consequently how a person's brain 'sees' the surroundings can cause a person's behaviour. However it may be possible to stop some of these behaviors by adapting a person's environment, just as you would for other disabilities. For instance replacing patterned curtains, carpets, wallpaper, clothes, bed spreads, cushions etc with plain ones.

Case study. Margaret

Margaret's husband, John, had called her Community Mental Health Nurse to ask for some advice. He was worried that Margaret had started to hallucinate because she was saying that she could see snakes in the bedroom. The nurse suggested to John that he reassure her that there were no snakes in the room and that it was only her imagination.

John called back a week later to say that this had not helped, so the nurse agreed to come over and have a word with Margaret. During the visit the nurse asked to see their bedroom, while in there the nurse noticed that the curtains had a long spiral pattern on them.

The nurse asked John if the curtains were new and he confirmed that they were. Consequently she suggested taking the curtains down and replacing them with plain ones. John was reluctant to do this but agreed that he would.

A while later the nurse called John to see how Margaret was getting on. John told her that the change in curtains had worked.

Other Reasons for Behaviour.

Although changes to the brain will inevitably have some affect on a person's behaviour, to only rely on this as an explanation would simplify the complexity of a person with dementia as a human being. Consequently it is important to consider other causes such as:

- **A person's past.** All of us are affected by our past, it gives us an insight into how to act in certain situations. Often a person with dementia will be significantly influenced by the role they played in their life, including their parental and occupational roles, as shown in the case study below. Some people with dementia may 'wander' around because they have always enjoyed walking.
- **Pain & discomfort.** When we need help because we feel unwell all we have to do is ask. However for people with dementia, because of problems with their speech, they may have to rely heavily on their behaviour.
- **Medication.** The side effects of a person's medication could be causing the behaviour.
- **Others.** Other people will influence a person's behaviour especially if they are asked to do something they can not do or are made to feel foolish or inadequate.
- **A person's surroundings**. A person's environment will influence their behaviour. For example loud noise could be a source of distress.

- **Emotional need.** Sometime people with dementia may refer to significant others in their life because they are trying to express a need. For example a person may be asking for their mother because they are lonely and need someone to comfort them? Or is a person asking to go to work because they are bored and want something to do?

Case study. Daniel

Daniel was 85 and visited a day care centre for people with dementia. The staff had very little information about Daniel's past, other then the fact that he had a brother who lived in Portugal. Often, after lunch, Daniel would start to move furniture around the dining room. When staff tried to intervene, Daniel would become aggressive.

Staff were becoming concerned about Daniel's behaviour and the manager of the home was considering moving him to another service. However the manager decided to contact Daniel's brother for advice.

During their conversation he mentioned that Daniel had been a furniture removal man in his twenties and this could possibly be the reason for his behaviour. It became obvious that Daniel was behaving this way because staff were stopping him from doing his job.

With this information staff would ask Daniel to move particular furniture that they had decided it was safe to do so. Although Daniel was occasionally aggressive it became less frequent.

Looking for Triggers.

When considering the reasons behind a person's behaviour it is worth thinking about what triggered or caused the behaviour. A trigger is something used to describe anything that causes a person's behaviour. This could include:

- Being in a noisy room.
- Another individual has shouted at the person
- The person with dementia does not know where they are.
- The person is asked to do something they can't do.

Writing a diary of the behaviours shown may allow a pattern to emerge of when each behaviour occurs.

In the next chapter the concept of person centered care is looked at and considered.

Chapter Five

Person Centred Care

This chapter will explore the concept of person centred care – a type of care that considers a number of factors that will influence a person other then just the brain damage.

What is person-centred care?

Person-centred care was developed by a number of individuals, including the late Professor Tom Kitwood & Professor Mary Marshall. They believed that too many care professionals focused heavily on the illness and not enough on the person and what they were going through. As a result they promoted support called person-centred care.

This concept is about recognising that a person with dementia is a person first and foremost. They may have dementia but this is only one of the many factors that need to be considered when supporting them.

See the diagram overleaf.

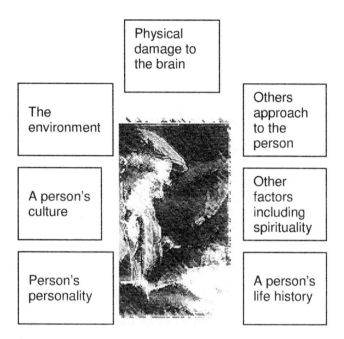

Person-centred care focuses on the wide range of needs a person with dementia has rather then just a set of symptoms that need to be treated.

Sometimes person-centred care is referred to as the new culture of care. This is to distinguish it from different types of care, known as the old culture.

What is the old culture of care?

This term refers to practices of care that developed in the old asylums and institutions. Asylums were buildings where people with dementia were often sent among with other social 'outcasts'. However these were not places of support.

An example of one such asylum was Bethlem Royal Hospital (Bedlam).In the 18th century it became famous for allowing visitors to pay to come and watch the 'patients' as a form of entertainment.

In these places people with dementia were seen as 'lunatics' and classed as 'insane'. It was even believed that people with dementia were unable to experience feelings of worth and well-being, because of damage to their brain. This meant that people did not consider what the person with dementia was feeling or going through and so it was thought unimportant to give quality care to people with dementia.

Examples of the old culture of care include:
- Not giving the person with dementia choices about what they would like to eat, what they would like to wear, what they would like to do etc.
- Treating the person with dementia as a child or a number.
- Moving a person with dementia like a piece of furniture or an object.
- Talking about the person with dementia in front of them as if they were not there.
- Going too fast for the person to understand.

- Ignoring the fact that a person with dementia has feelings and emotions.
- Not considering how a person's life history and life experiences will affect them.

The late professor Tom Kitwood called these practices Malignant Social Psychology. He deliberately used the term malignant

In the 1980's Care in the Community was developed by the Conservative party. Its aim was to help people with mental health problems, by removing them from institutions, and caring for them in their own homes. However despite closures of many of these large institutions a negative view of people with dementia still remains.

An example of this is the negative language used by some professionals and the media to describe people with dementia, such as:

- Demented
- Sufferer
- Difficult
- Awkward
- Burden
- Living funeral
- Deterioration

It is true that some people with dementia may suffer and may feel a burden, but there will be times when a person with dementia can feel happy and useful.

"We still have a laugh".

"They can't speak up for themselves".

Using the term *sufferer* gives the opinion that people are constantly suffering which is not the case for a lot of people. Also the term evokes sympathy, feeling sorry for the person. Most people with dementia do not want people without dementia to be sympathetic. Instead they want us to be empathic, to try and understand what they are going through.

There will be times when a person deteriorates because of their illness. Even so, there will be times when a person can have periods of improvement because of the positive care provided.

These words provide us with a very limited view of people with dementia, one that is still trapped in the old culture of care. Neither do they hold much hope for the person themselves or their families. These words paint a very bleak view of the future and whilst there will be very difficult times for many people there will also be positive times during the experience of dementia. The table below shows some of the differences between the old and new language.

Old language	New Language
Wandering	**Exploring, looking for something or someone.**
Agitated	**Feeling frightened, scared.**
Demented	**Person with dementia.**

However it is not only the language of the asylums that still exist. Many professionals' views of people with dementia are still deeply routed in the asylum.

An example of this is the professional's decision not to tell people with dementia their diagnosis. According to a report by the National Audit Office (2007) people with dementia in the UK are often not told, unlike in other European countries. Many medical professionals make their decision not to tell the person based on their knowledge about dementia and not on their knowledge about the person. For example they may believe that people with dementia will not be able to cope with the reality or will simply forget or not understand. This is the case for some people with dementia but certainly not all. Especially now more people are seeking diagnosis from the medical profession earlier due to increased public awareness about dementia.

For those people who could understand their diagnosis, being left in the dark will add to feelings of paranoia and will prevent a person being offered choices about support and treatment (such as counselling, links to a local Alzheimer's Society branch or a support group), being able to resolve financial matters and discuss with others the future before it is late. So the reality is a person's choice to know is taken out of their hands, and consequently reflects treatment of people with cancer thirty-years ago. The person is forgotten in favour of the illness.

"The paper version of the person seems to have become more important than the one with the heart beat...when CSCI come they want to look at the care plan rather than the person".

Kitwood introduced the concept of person-centred care to try and prevent such occurrences. He believed that all people with dementia should be valued and not treated like second-class citizens. He strongly argued that if people with dementia are given the opportunity to grow in confidence and feel good about themselves then this will help them cope through the journey of their illness.

Person-centred care differs significantly in its views about dementia to the traditional views of dementia as shown in the diagram below.

Traditional view of dementia	Person-centred view.
Dementia – any form of insanity characterised by the failure or loss of mental powers, the organic deterioration of intelligence, memory and orientation, often with advanced age. Chambers Dictionary	Dementia is a disability. The impact this disability has on a person depends on how well we compensate for it.
Not a lot can be done to help a person with dementia other then waiting for a cure or providing for their physical needs.	People with dementia can still have a good quality of life if we focus on a person's different needs.

Behaviours are a symptom of dementia.	All behaviour has meaning. Behaviours are a form of communication. We need to try and understand what the person is telling us through their behaviour.
Dementia is an experience of constant loss	People with dementia, no matter how late on in the illness, still have strengths and abilities.
People with dementia are not like us because they have an "organic mental disorder".	People with dementia are the same as us – they are equal members of society.
Health professionals are the experts	People with dementia and their families are experts. They are living with the illness.

The concepts behind Person-centred care.

Person centred care stresses people should be allowed to live a 'normal' life without being constantly reminded of their limitations and losses. This can be done by

- **Focusing on how a person's past life will effect them now during their illness.**
  When we are able to build a detailed picture of the person with dementia this often proves an invaluable tool in both effective communication and person-centered care. It enables us to begin building a good relationship with the person by providing us with a greater understanding of the individual behind the condition.

72

- **Enabling choice.**

  The reality is that people are no given the opportunity to make decisions. Often this is done for them because it is believed that a person can't make their own decisions. There will be certain decisions that carers and professional will need to make, but if a person looses all control then this will undoubtedly have a negative affect on them. Therefore it is important to consider how to use skills effectively to enable people to take an active role in their care.

- **Maintaining Identity.**

  This refers to who the person is as an individual. Consider the building blocks of who the person with dementia is and how they see themselves.

- **Observing Dignity.**

  This is strongly linked to the way we feel about ourselves. People who have dementia may often feel that their privacy and dignity is threatened. This needs to be respected.

- **Recognising Culture.**

  All of us have a cultural identity. This is an identity that a person shares with a group who follow similar cultural practices including holidays and customs. For example if you were aware that a person with dementia had certain cultural beliefs about food it would be important to respect that when providing their meals.

- **Respecting Spiritual beliefs.**

  This can mean different things for different people. Spirituality can be very important for a person with dementia because it can give support and a sense of purpose

- **Considering Emotional needs.**
  People with dementia do not lose their feelings or emotions. People with dementia still need to be able to experience the feelings of joy, self-worth, fulfilment and love.

- **Supporting Social Needs.**
  People with dementia still need to relate and have relationships with others. Not having this in a person with dementia's life can lead to them becoming isolated.

- **Encouraging communication.**
  Because of the difficulties faced by a person with dementia it can be wrongly assumed that a person can't communicate and consequently other people may stop talking with the person with dementia or they may no longer involve them in conversations. This can have detrimental affect on a person with dementia's health and mental well-being.

Criticism of Person centered care

There have been a number of issues raised about person centered care. This includes:

- The amount of time needed to practice this type of care is considerable and so is not achievable in health care setting where there are large numbers of people with dementia.

- Carers may be blamed for a person with dementia's decline because person centered care was not practiced.

- Without the medical field the anti-dementia drugs (chapter six) would never have been developed.

- The terms used by Kitwood and others can be jargonistic and so can cause confusion for staff about how to achieve this type of care.

Despite these criticisms it cannot be denied that person centred care has provided us with a different view about what is important in the care of people with dementia.

In the next chapter we look at different drug treatments.

Chapter Six

Drug Treatments.

This sixth chapter will consider some of the different medications that people with dementia can use including the anti dementia drugs. Although this chapter focuses on drug treatment it also indicates that this is not the only form of treatment for people with dementia. Consequently other forms of treatment are looked at in chapters seven and eight.

There is currently no cure for dementia. Once a brain cell has been damaged or destroyed it cannot be repaired. However there are a number of drugs that can potentially help with some of the symptoms experienced by a person with dementia.

The next diagram shows some of the different categories of drugs that people with dementia may be given.

See diagram overleaf

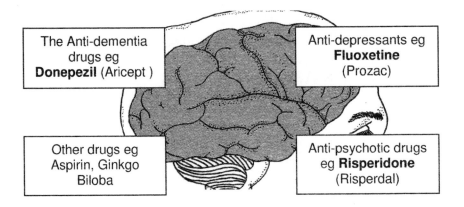

The Anti-dementia drugs eg **Donepezil** (Aricept)

Anti-depressants eg **Fluoxetine** (Prozac)

Other drugs eg Aspirin, Ginkgo Biloba

Anti-psychotic drugs eg **Risperidone** (Risperdal)

The anti- dementia drugs.

There are a group of drugs, called the anti dementia drugs or acetylcholinesterase inhibitors, that can help with some of the symptoms of Alzheimer's disease in some individuals.

Currently there are three anti-dementia drugs. These are:

- Donepezil (Aricept)
- Rivastigmine (Exelon)
- Galantamine (Reminyl)

Studies have been undertaken into the use of the anti-dementia drugs in other causes of dementia including dementia with lewy bodies and Vascular dementia. However these drugs are usually only used for people with Alzheimer's disease and not the other types of dementia.

QUESTION. WHY DO DRUGS HAVE TWO NAMES?

Most drugs have two names. The generic name and the brand name, in brackets. This refers to the medical name and the name the manufactures call the drug

How do the anti-dementia drugs work?

There are more then a 100 billion cells in a person's brain. These cells are called neurons. These neurons communicate with one another by sending chemical messages across a small gap.

Acetylcholine is one of these chemicals that crosses this tiny space. (This chemical is needed to help us learn, remember information and it is also involved in movement). While this is happening, an enzyme, called Acetylcholinesterase, breaks down some of the Acetylcholine so that it can be used again.

The anti-dementia drugs work by stopping the Acetylcholinesterase from eating the Acetylcholine. As a result these drugs boost the amount of the chemical within a person with Alzheimer's brain.

The following diagrams show what happens in a person's brain, a person with Alzheimer's brain and finally how the anti-dementia drugs work.

Fig 1.

A person without Alzheimer's.

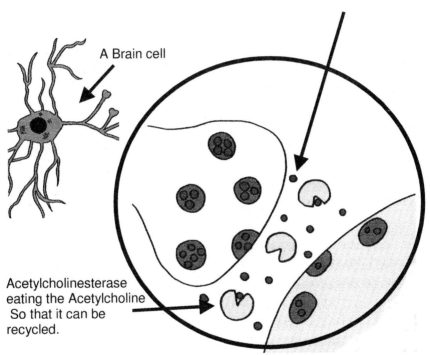

Acetylcholine crossing the gap between two brain cells.

A Brain cell

Acetylcholinesterase eating the Acetylcholine So that it can be recycled.

****

Fig 2.

A person with Alzheimer's disease.

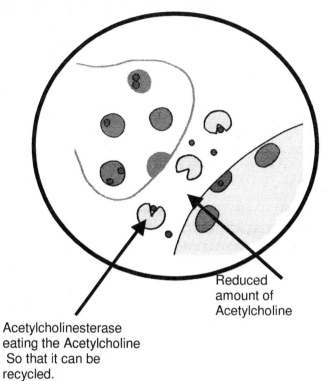

Reduced
amount of
Acetylcholine

Acetylcholinesterase
eating the Acetylcholine
So that it can be
recycled.

****

Fig 3.

With the anti-dementia drugs.

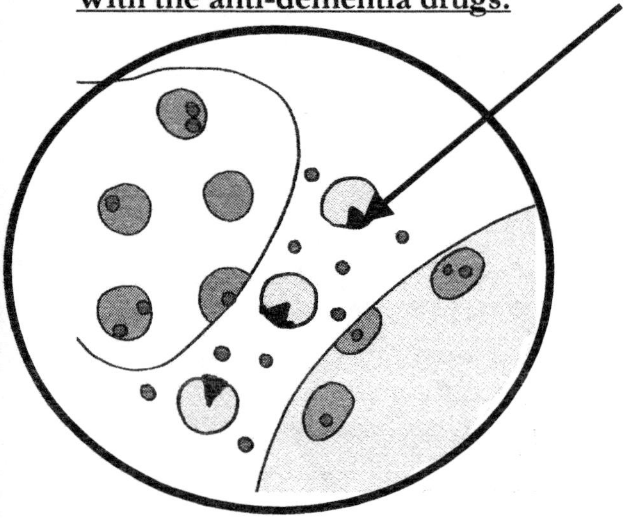

The drug blocks the Acetylcholinesterase and so stops it from breaking down the Acetylcholine. This then increases the amount of Acetylcholine in a person with Alzheimer's brain.

****

Memantine (Ebixa).

There is another type of drug called Memantine (Ebixa) that can help people with Alzheimer's in the later stages of dementia. This drug works differently to the above the anti-dementia drugs by stopping a chemical called Glutamate, which can cause damage to the brain cells.

However none of these drugs stop the disease and eventually, as more brain cells are killed by the plaques and tangles, the drugs will no longer be helpful.

Case Study. Mrs. Kinson

Mrs. Kinson had lived in a care home for older people with dementia for 3 months. The staff and her GP believed that she had adjusted well to her new environment. Mrs. Kinson was prescribed Rivastigmine (Exelon) by her GP and soon after she regained some of her lost skills. As result she decided that she did not want to be in a home for people with dementia. When her family told her that her home had been sold to fund her care she became very angry at her family telling them they should have never put her into 'such a place'.

Considerations include when should a person be given an anti-dementia drug, when should they stop taking the drug and do the positives outweigh the side effects of the anti-dementia medication. (The increase of acetylcholine caused by the anti dementia drugs not only affects the brain but can also influence other parts of the body such as the stomach. Consequently common side effects can include diarrhea and vomiting. If there are concerns about the side effects of any drug a person's doctor should be contacted).

Nice

In 2001 (NICE) the National Institute for Health and Clinical excellence (a governmental advisory body) approved prescription of these drugs on the National Health Service. However in late 2006 NICE changed their advice claiming that, from the evidence collected, the anti dementia drugs did not make enough of a difference to people with Alzheimer's disease to warrant the cost to the NHS. Consequently it has advised that people with Alzheimer's disease in the early and later stages of the illness are no longer to be prescribed these medications on the NHS. People in the moderate stage of Alzheimer's can be prescribed the anti – dementia drugs by the NHS. However it is questionable, by this point, if the drugs are of any benefit. Doctors have also been advised not to prescribe the drug Ebixa due to it not being cost effective.

Despite this advice from NICE doctors are still able to make considerations based on their view of what is in the best interests of their patients. However this decision will depend on a number of factors including available funding.

People with dementia can still purchase this medication privately, however many have argued that people should have not to pay for this treatment and secondly the majority of people with dementia are of pensionable age and therefore may struggle to pay. In response to this different drug companies and the Alzheimer's society challenged this decision in the High Court. Nevertheless in August 2007 the High Court ruled in favor of NICE.

More information about NICE and this ruling can be found at **www.nice.org.uk.**

Alternatives.

As a consequence of the ruling regarding the anti dementia drugs it is possible that more people will turn to other medication for help with symptoms.

One such treatment that could possible help is Ginkgo Biloba. This is a drug made from the leaves of the Maidenhair Tree.

Also different vitamins have been looked at including vitamin B supplements to see if they are beneficial for people with dementia, but as with the Ginkgo more research is needed. It is important to speak to a person's doctor before taking such treatments.

Aspirin

This commonly used drug is often used for pain relief and to reduce the development of blood clots and consequently strokes. People with vascular dementia may already be taking aspirin to treat their existing vascular problems.

The use of Aspirin and other Non-Steroidal Anti-Inflammatory drugs such as ibuprofen may also help people with dementia. However these drugs can cause side effects such as stomach ulcers and so should not be used as a way of trying to stop getting dementia.

Anti-Psychotic drugs.

Another group of drugs, called the anti-psychotics, are mainly used to help people with schizophrenia. These drugs are also used to help people with dementia who are perceived to be 'agitated' or 'aggressive' or paranoid. The anti-psychotics (also known as major tranquillizers) are a large group of drugs that include:

- Chlorpromazine (Largactil)
- Risperidone (Risperdal)
- Haloperidol (Haldol)

These drugs can be helpful for a number of people with dementia, yet there have been a number of arguments that stress the need for caution when giving such drugs to people with dementia.

Firstly it has been suggested that the anti psychotics are to often used as the first response to challenging behaviour rather then looking at other alternatives first, such as identifying triggers (See chapter four). Furthermore it has been argued that these drugs do not actually find the reason for the behaviour but instead only mask the problems by sedating the person.

Secondly, research has suggested that there is an over reliance on the use of the anti-psychotic drugs for people with dementia living in care. In the US there was great concern about this, which led to the introduction of the Omnibus Budget Reconciliation Act (1987). This piece of legislation aimed to prevent the over prescription of these drugs.

Thirdly, people with dementia may be left on this medication for longer then necessary. Consequently this can increase the risk of a person experiencing side effects. For instance some of the older anti-psychotics have the potential to cause Parkinson type symptoms in a person such as problems with mobility, thinking and facial expression.

Drug name	Possible side effects
Chlorpromazine (Largactil)	Drowsiness blurring of vision, fainting.
Risperidone (Risperdal)	Insomnia, anxiety, agitation, headache, drowsiness, dizziness, weight gain, rash, thirst.
Haloperidol (Haldol)	Dry mouth, blurred vision, difficulty in passing urine, appetite loss.

Finally research has indicted that these drugs can actually be very harmful if given to a person with dementia with lewy bodies.

As a consequence of the issues concerned it is beneficial if collaboration between medication and other factors are considered as indicated in the case study of Mr. Hutchinson, see overleaf.

Case study. Mr Hutchinson.

Mr. Hutchinson had lived in a Nursing home for two years. Mr. Hutchinson had shown signs of aggression over the two years but recently this had increased. His Doctor assessed him and decided that he would benefit from a small dose of Risperidone, twice daily.

This seemed to reduce the level of aggression shown by Mr. Hutchinson but staff reported that he was having trouble with his balance and had fallen twice. Mr. Hutchinson's wife was concerned that her husband would seriously hurt himself as a result of the falls and consequently his medication was reduced to once daily.

Although Mr. Hutchinson was no longer physically aggressive he started to become verbally abusive to the staff. Rather then increasing the dose of Risperidone again the manager of the home decided to undertake external staff training that looked at ways of understanding the reasons behind the verbal outbursts and how to try and handle Mr. Hutchinson when he became angry.

Anti- Parkinson drugs

A person with dementia would usually only receive these types of drugs if they had Parkinson's disease as well as their dementia. Parkinson's disease affects a person's brain by reducing a chemical called **DOPAMINE**. Dopamine has many functions in the brain including helping with our movement. A lack of dopamine in the brain results in people having problems with movement, involuntary shakes, rigidity & slowness of thinking. People with Parkinson's may be given drug treatment to help relieve some of the symptoms of Parkinson's disease. However they do not cure the disease. Instead the anti-Parkinson drugs work by either:

- Replacing the missing dopamine. A drug called Benserazide hydrochloride (Madopar) does this.
- Copying the actions of dopamine, such as Bromocriptine (Parlodel)
- Stopping the break down of dopamine, such as Selegiline hydrochloride (Carbex).

The next chapter looks at the different roles of people who can help those with dementia and their families.

****

Chapter Seven

Support Systems

There are a number of sources of support available for people with dementia and their families/carers. Nevertheless these may be difficult to find or access. Additionally numerous barriers may prevent access including lack of time, an unsuitable location or a person may simply be too exhausted to try and access a service. Consequently this chapter aims to provide information about a number of sources of potential support and details of where to get help.

Health and Social Care

The main areas of support come from Health and Social care. This care can be provided through orgnnisations such as the NHS or Social Services, through charities or independent providers.

Health care refers to the physical and emotional care a person with dementia receives. This can include both primary and secondary care. Primary care refers to support received in the community – this is often the initial care form a GP. Secondary care is for people with dementia that require further support. For example the GP may decide that a person needs to go to hospital to see a specialist.

The term social care covers a wide range of services that can support people's various needs including, housing and accommodation, daily living skills and emotional.

Some of the different services provided by health and social care are shown in the following 2 diagrams.

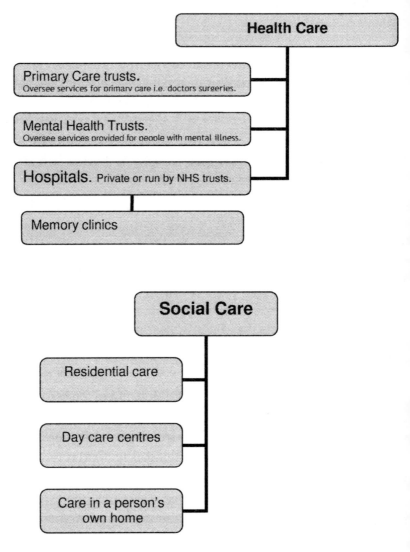

Support from Health Care

Health care usually involves support from:

A General Practitioner (GP). For the majority of people with dementia and their carers this is usually the first port of call to try and discover an explanation for symptoms.

> **FACT**
>
> **There are GP's across England that have a specialist knowledge in dementia. These are known as GP with Special Interest or GPwSI.**

A GP may make a diagnosis based on the information they have and will then continue to monitor a person during their experience of dementia.

Alternatively a GP may refer a person to a specialist. This could be either an old age Psychiatrist if the person is over 65, or a Neurologist, usually if the person is below 65. A diagnosis of dementia can also be made by a Geriatrician, if the person is admitted to hospital.

Diagnosis usually occurs after a person's medical history and lifestyle have been considered, and other possible causes have been ruled out and relevant tests have been undertaken.

These tests can include brain scans, such as a CT (computerised tomography) or an MRI (Magnetic resonance imaging). Other tests can include memory tests, such as the Mini Mental State Examination (MMSE) or the Addenbrooke's Cognitive Examination (ACE).

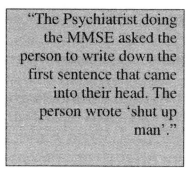
"The Psychiatrist doing the MMSE asked the person to write down the first sentence that came into their head. The person wrote 'shut up man'."

These tests involve asking a person with dementia a number of questions to try and assess their ability to recall recent information.

GP's may also make a referral to one of the following services for diagnosis and treatment, depending on availability in the area.

Community mental health team for older people. There are a number of community mental health teams (CMHT) for older adults around the country. These are group of different professionals including psychiatrists; clinical psychologists and community mental health nurses that provide psychological support for people with severe mental illness. Although some CMHT's provide support for people with dementia, this is not the case for all teams.

A memory clinic. This is also a team of specialists however, rather then focusing on a wide range of mental illnesses they specialise in dementia and other causes of severe memory loss. They are usually located within an NHS trust

Case Study: Mark West

Mark is a 67 year-old man with vascular dementia, who has a high level of awareness about his difficulties. The family GP had monitored his diagnosis and consequent treatment. However Mark's wife became concerned about her husbands well being after he started to talk about suicide and so informed Marks's GP. After seeing Mark, the GP referred him to the local Community Mental Health Team, where Mark saw an old age Psychiatrist and a Community Mental Health Nurse.

An assessment was undertaken and it was concluded that Mark was at a high risk of attempting suicide. Consequently It was decided that he would benefit from taking anti-depressants. It was also suggested that Mark spend time on a mental health ward to monitor his progress.

Nurses. There are a wide-range of nurses who can support people with dementia. This includes

"The nurses never actually spoke to us – not like people. All they could ever say was 'are you all right'? When you told them no they didn't want to hear".

District Nurses. These visit people with dementia in their own homes or care homes to provide various physical nursing care.

Community Mental Health Nurses (also called Community psychiatric nurses, CPN). This type of nurse provides advice and assessments about mental health care for people with dementia at home or in care homes.

Registered Mental Nurses (RMN). They will care for a person with dementia if they are is admitted to a mental health hospital or ward.

Admiral Nurses. These individuals specialise in working with people with dementia and their carers. They can provide information, practical advice and help other professionals to deliver positive care. Admiral Nurses Direct is an advice and support line and can be called on **0845 257 9406** or emailed on direct@fordementia.org.uk.

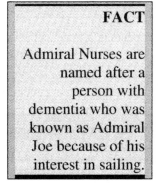

FACT

Admiral Nurses are named after a person with dementia who was known as Admiral Joe because of his interest in sailing.

There are a number of Admiral nurses services around the country including the Midlands, Manchester and the South East. For details in your area you can look on the *For Dementia* website at:

www.fordementia.org.uk

Support from Social Care

Social Care for people with dementia and their carers is provided by either by Local Authorities or through independent organisations or charities.

Local Authorities will use guidelines to assess whether or not a person is eligible for help from Adult Social Services.
This assessment will usually be undertaken by a social worker. If it is felt that a person is eligible then the social services department will arrange any services that the assessment decides are required. This can include support through domiciliary care, day care services, self-directed support etc.

If a person is not eligible then social services should signpost the person onto other organisations that may help.

Self Directed Support. Local Authorities provide funding to pay for some people's social care support. Until recently people were not told about how much this support cost and were not fully involved in the process, known as care management. However Self Directed Support encourages a person to lead the whole process, rather then be led by a social worker, and to have control about how their money is used.

A person can ask anyone to help them with the Self Directed Support Process including their family and friends and social worker etc.

However to receive Self Directed Support a person would still need to meet the social services eligibility criteria. Currently not all

Local Authorities are providing Self Directed Support.

Domiciliary care. This is support that is provided for people with dementia in their own homes. This can include a wide range of support from helping a person to get dressed to actual nursing care. Social Services or indpendet providers can provide domiciliary care.

Many of the domiciliary services are represented by an organization called the United Kingdom Home Care Association (UKHCA) that aims to provide quality care to people living in their own homes. All members of the UKHCA agree to follow a code of practice that promotes quality care.

Daycare services. This includes day centers or day clubs that can provide people with dementia an opportunity to meet with others, usually in a fixed environment such as a community centre or a church hall. (Moore et al 2004). Social Services, Charities and indepdnet providers can provide daycare.

 One of the many factors day care services have to consider is the issue of transport i.e. how the person with dementia travels from their own home to the centre and back.

The Community Transport Association is a national organisation regarding community and voluntary transport who can often help services with these issues. (www.communitytransport.com)

Respite. This is a period of relief, for a carer, from caring. It can come in the form of a relief carer, an individual who supports a person with dementia in his or her own home, or from a care home. A short stay in a care home can be beneficial for a carer however it can prove unsettling for a person with dementia because of its unfamiliarity.

Respite can be provided by Social Services or through an organisation such as Cross Roads- caring for carers provides relief carers.

Care homes can provide care for people with dementia of any age. However there are only a few care homes especially for people with dementia below 65. (The Alzheimer's Society provides a list of services for younger people on their website at www.alzheimers.org.uk/ypwd).

Care homes can provide support either with or without nursing care. When considering a care home it is worth reading the inspection report, this can be provided either by the home or can be found on the CSCI website: www.csci.org.uk.

Sheltered Housing usually consists of purpose-built environments, e.g. a set of apartments that have a warden and specialist equipment to provide assistance, if needed. Organisations, such as the Elderly Accommodation Council can help (Advice line. 020 7820 1343).

'Meals on Wheels' deliver hot or cold meals to a person's house. Social services usually provide this though a charity such as the Women's Royal Voluntary Service (telephone 029 2073 9000) or a catering firm.

Services provided by social care are inspected by the Commission for Social Care Inspection (CSCI). The Commission inspects all social care services including statutory, private and voluntary.

Also those who work in Social care and regulated by the General Social Care Council. This organisation was set up to help services provide quality care.

Jargon

In the world of dementia care there is lots of jargon and acronyms. The table below summarizes some of these.

CMHT	Community Mental Health Team
CPN	Community Psychiatric Nurse
MMSE	Mini Mental State Examination
RMN	Registered Mental Nurse
MRI	Magnetic resonance imaging
PCT	Primary Care Trusts
CSCI	Commission for Social Care Inspection

Support from dementia care charities and organisations.

As the name suggests voluntary services are provided by volunteers or organisations that do not make a profit i.e. charities. Although a number of charities rely heavily on volunteers to survive many national charities also employ people to help with the development and stability of these organisations.

Charities are regulated by a governing body called The Charity Commission.

The Alzheimer's Society.

This charity provides services for anyone who has been affected by any type of dementia, including people with dementia, families, carers and professionals.

They have been a key force in battling for change in government policies to provide better care for people with dementia and their carers.

The organisation itself was set up by two carers back in the 1970's. The society provides help nationally through the Alzheimer's Help line (0845 300 0336) and through branches of the Alzheimer's Society. These branches can be found around the county and local support. This can come in many forms including:

- Day clubs/ centers.

- Support groups for carers and people with dementia

- Advice sheets including information on benefits, different types of dementia, where and how to get help.

• Training for people with dementia and their carers.

• Publications about different issues faced by people with dementia and their carers.

Alzheimer Scotland

In Scotland people with dementia, their carers and families are supported by an organization called **Alzheimer's Scotland** - Action on Dementia.

Alzheimer's disease International

Alzheimer's disease International is an umbrella organisation of Alzheimer's associations around the world, which offer support and information to people with dementia and their caregivers.

Contact Details
Alzheimer's Society, Devon House, 58 St Katharine's Way. London E1W 1JX
020 7423 3500
Email
enquiries@alzheimers.org.uk
www.alzheimers.org.uk/

Alzheimer Scotland, 22 Drumsheugh Gardens, Edinburgh. EH3 7RN
Phone: 0131 243 1453.
E-mail: alzheimer@alzscot.org.
www.alzscot.org.uk

Alzheimer's disease International
http://www.alz.co.uk/

The Picks Disease Support Group 8 Brooksby Close, Oadby, Leicester. LE2 5AB
Phone: 0116 271 1414
info@pdsg.org.uk
www.pdsg.org.uk

The Picks Disease Support Group.

This charity was established for carers and people with the Fronto-temporal dementia's .

CJD Support Network.
PO Box 346, Market Drayton,
Shropshire TF9 4WN
Phone: 01630 673 993
www.cjdsupport.net

CJD Support Network.
This network of families and volunteers supports people with CJD and their families.

Lewy Body Society
Holland House, 10 Chestnut Drive, Hatfield Heath
Herts CM22 7EZ
info@lewybody.org.
www.lewybody.org

Lewy Body Society
This is a UK charity providing support for people with dementia with lewy bodies.

The Alzheimer's Research Trust.
The Stables, Station Road, Great Shelford,
Cambridge. CB22 5LR
Phone: 01223 843899
enquiries@alzheimers-research.org.uk
www.alzheimers-research.org.uk

The Alzheimer's research Trust.
This registered charity undertakes research into dementia, including improving the accuracy of diagnosis. However it relies solely on donations.

The Clive project
PO Box 315, Witney,
Oxfordshire. OX28 1ZN
Phone: 01993 776295
mail@thecliveproject.org.uk

The Clive project
This service cares for and supports younger people with dementia and their family and friends.

Crossroads Association
10 Regent Place
Rugby
Warwickshire. CV21 2PN
Phone: 0845 450 0350

Crossroads.
This service gives carers the opportunity for periods of respite.

Other Organisations.

Dementia Services Development Centres (DSDC)

These are organsiations across the counrty that provide services and information about dementia inlcuding services available in that area.

To find your nearest DSDC, go to **www.dsdcengland.org.uk**

www.dasninternational.org

DASNI: Dementia Advocacy and Support Network International

This is an excellent website run by people with dementia, with many personal stories.

At dementia
9 Newarke Street,
Leicester. LE1 5SN
Phone: 0116 257 5017
info@trentdsdc.org.uk
www.atdementia.org.uk

At dementia

This web site is run by Trent Dementia Services Development Centre and provides information about assertive technologies, including what they are and where to get them.

Chapter eight examines some of the different therapies available for people with dementia.

Chapter Eight.

Therapies

This chapter examines some of the different therapies available for people with dementia, including occupational therapy, physiotherapy and complimentary therapies.

There are a number of therapies that may be offered to a person with dementia, or their carers, after a diagnosis. These include:

Occupational therapy.

An occupational therapist (OT) is a person trained in occupational therapy. Their role in helping people with dementia involves helping the person to maintain as much independence as possible.

"Can any of the things be changed? How can they be changed? Whose help do I need to change them? The list goes on and I am getting bored with it."

This can be done:

• By assessing a person's needs.

• Through helping with daily living activities such as washing and dressing.

• By suggesting equipment that can be used by a person or their carer to help the person remain at home for as long as possible.

• By suggesting activities and exercises that can be undertaken to maintain a person with dementia's physical health.

More Occupational Services are being provided for people with dementia. To find out if an OT would be beneficial a person could ask their GP for a referral or they could contact their local occupational therapy department. This department could be based either in a local hospital or with the local social services. The local telephone directory will have these numbers. Alternatively the British Association of Occupational Therapist could be contacted on 020 7357 6480

Physiotherapy.

Physiotherapists can help people with dementia with physical problems enabling the person to maintain or improve their movement. Furthermore they can offer advice about body positioning to help with eating, washing and walking.

However people with dementia are not always given the opportunity for physiotherapy. This may be because it is believed that the person will not be able to follow the therapist's instructions and advice. Greater concentration is given to supporting a family carer by giving advice about keeping them mobile and healthy.

There are a number of physiotherapists who specialise in working with people with mental health problems, including dementia.

The Chartered Society of Physiotherapists in Mental Healthcare c/o Caroline Griffiths Physiotherapy Dept Warneford hospital Oxford, OX3

01865 223811

"Personally I don't get it. When did talking ever change anything?"

"It helped me to see that I am not the only one. This knowledge in itself gave me a sense of comfort"

Talking therapies.

This term covers a wide range of therapies undertaken with people with dementia and their families including support groups, Psychotherapy and counselling.

Although these types of support are still limited, in particular for people with dementia, there is growing recognition of the benefits in particular of support groups.

These are organised groups where people affected by dementia can share their experiences and provide one another with advice or support.

Originally these groups were run for families and carers. However more groups are being offered for people with dementia, through the Alzheimer's Society and projects such as the Dementia Voice Project.

Physiotherapy.

Physiotherapists can help people with dementia with physical problems enabling the person to maintain or improve their movement. Furthermore they can offer advice about body positioning to help with eating, washing and walking.

The Chartered Society of Physiotherapists Physiotherapy Dept Warneford hospital Oxford, OX3 01865 223811

However people with dementia are not always given the opportunity for physiotherapy. This may be because it is believed that the person will not be able to follow the therapist's instructions and advice. Greater concentration is given to supporting a family carer by giving advice about keeping them mobile and healthy.

There are a number of physiotherapists who specialise in working with people with mental health problems, including dementia.

Complementary therapies

As well as treatment through medication more people are turning to complementary therapies as a way of easing some of the symptoms of dementia. There is an abundance of research into these therapies including:

Acupuncture

This therapy originates from ancient China, which involves placing needles into specific parts of a person's body. Some research has indicated that this may be helpful for people with dementia.

Contact details.

The British Medical Acupuncture Society
12 Marbury House
Higher Whitley
Warrington. WA4 4QW
01925 730727

Aromatherapy & Massage.

This involves using therapeutic oils to help reduce anxiety and stress in people with dementia. These oils, taken from plants, such as tea-tree oil, are used

International Federation of Aromatherapists
61-63 Churchfield Road,
Acton, London
W3 6AY
020 8992 9605

through massage onto a person's skin. Alternatively these oils can be placed in a burner or a diffuser to release a smell.

Validation therapy.

This technique was developed by Naomi Feil. The therapy acknowledges the person's feelings and accepts their beliefs even if they contradict our own. For example if a person with dementia thought their mother was still alive the validation approach would try to find out from the person with dementia why they were asking for their mother, i.e. is the person feeling lonely, do they need someone to confide in or to gain comfort from etc.

Snoezelen.

This involves creating a multi-sensory environment for people with dementia i.e. different things to look at and feel. Items that can be used include bubble tubes, fibre optics and light projectors. Although some people with dementia may find this a relaxing experience, others may find the experience distressing because a snoezelen room can look very unusual.

Reminiscence therapy.

Reminiscence refers to remembering events from the past. This can be very beneficial for people with dementia due to their ability to recall long term memories easier then short term memories. Reminiscence can occur through out the day with people with dementia either by talking about the past or by using objects from the past such as old photographs. Some care homes have developed reminiscence rooms to assist bringing back old memories and encourage conversation. However reminiscence can cause people distress especially if negative memories are recalled and no support is given to cope with these. Furthermore many people with dementia can start to 'live in the past'. For example the person with dementia may be 85 years old but they believe that they are 22. If a person is living in the past, it will seem unusual to them if you start asking questions such as 'do you remember using this?' or 'what job did you have?" This is because they may believe that they are still employed or still using those items.

Music therapy
Music is a powerful tool that is used to help people with dementia to build on their social skills and evoke memories from the past.

Dance therapy.
Dance therapy started as a way to support traumatised soldiers returning from World War 2. Since then it has been used for many conditions including dementia. Dancing is thought to help people with dementia, not only because of the physical exercise, but also emotionally because of the contact shared through dancing with others.

Sonas aPc
This is an approach in the care of older people who have communication difficulty, especially those who have dementia. It is the result of an initiative taken by the Sisters of Charity (RSCs) in 1990 and involves supporting people with dementia in a group through communication, music and stimulation of the senses.

Sonas aPc
St Mary's
201 Merrion Road
Dublin 4
Ireland
www.sonasapc.ie

110

Attachment therapy.

This type of therapy looks at providing people with dementia items to help them feel safe and at ease. One such example includes doll therapy. The use of dolls or soft toys may be seen by some as patronising to people with dementia. However growing evidence suggests that for some people such items can be a source of comfort. All of us, with or without dementia, have items of comfort that we turn to when needed.

The next chapter will focus on financial support and benefits.

Chapter Nine

Financial Support and Legislation.

People with dementia and their carers may be entitled to a range of benefits. This chapter will explore some of these benefits and provide sources of contact. However regulations on benefits do change so it is important to seek further advice from the contacts given.

Finally this chapter looks at some of the legislation that may be relevant to people with dementia and their families.

Scores of people with dementia, and their carers, find sorting through the maze of benefits feels like an uphill struggle. For many people in the early stages of dementia, worry about their financial affairs can cause extra stress and can result in people not claiming the benefits they are entitled to.

The benefits system is a complicated procedure and often people do miss out. It is not helped by the fact that the Department of Work and Pensions has no obligation to inform people about the different benefits. Further confusion can arise as different benefits are assessed by different organisations. For example an application for a benefit called the Attendance Allowance is undertaken by the Department of Work and Pensions where as a claim for council tax benefit is processed by the local authorities.

To try and make it easier it is worth thinking about benefits as a number of floors reached by sets of stairs. In this way hopefully any potential benefits will not be missed.

This includes
benefits that are non-means
tested – such as the Attendance
Allowance - and are tax free.

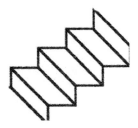

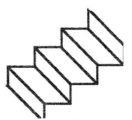

. Based on income and capital these are also means tested
benefits . ie)Pension credit.

.

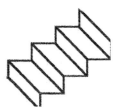

This first level is means tested according to
National contributions

First Floor benefits – Income replacement benefits

To be entitled to these benefits a person will not be working –
hence the name income replacement benefits. These benefits are
means tested. This means that a person's, and their partners,
income, contribution to National Insurance and savings will be
considered when deciding on the entitlement.

These first floor benefits include:

Carers allowance. This can be paid to carers of people with dementia who are caring for at least 35 hours a week. The person being cared for also needs to receive the attendance allowance, or disability living allowance at an appropriate rate. This can be complex and it may affect the amount of money the person with dementia is receiving so advice should be sought from one of the organisations listed later in the chapter.

State-Retirement Pension. A person is entitled to a state pension if they are of pensioable age (65 for men and between 60-65 for women, although this is changing in 2010) and they or their partner have contributed to national insurance.

Bereavement benefit. This can be claimed by widows or widowers who are below pensionable age and are over 45. Also the person should not have any children who are dependent on them. If the person does have a dependent then they would be entitled to Widows benefit.

Usually people cannot claim more then one of these benefits – for example if a person is receiving their state retirement pension they may not get carers allowance. Although it is worth applying for a number of these benefits as the person should be entitled to the highest paid benefit.

Second Floor benefits.
Second Floor benefits do not depend on national insurance contributions. Instead it is means tested by looking at a person's income or capital.

These benefits include:

Pension Credit. This benefits involves providing extra money each week for everyone aged 60 and over to guarantee a minimum level of income. The credit is at a higher level then the basic state retirement pension and considers a person's current weekly income.

Pension credit has two parts called savings credit and guarantee credit.

(i) The guarantee credit applies if a person is 60 or over This could help a single person whose weekly income is less then £124.05 or a couple whose weekly income is less then £189.35. If a person has a large amount of savings they may not receive this credit but it is still worth applying, just in case.

(ii) The savings credit applies to people who are over 65 and have a higher weekly income then the State Retirement Pension. The amount of money received can be potentially increased if a person is a carer or is severely disabled.

Housing benefit. This benefit helps individuals who are tenants to pay for rent. It is assessed according to a number of factors including income and the amount of rent being charged. If a person receives the guarantee part of the pension credit then they may get all of their rent paid.

Council Tax benefit. This benefit can help with part or all of the payments towards council tax. Once again if a person receives the guarantee part of the pension credit then they may get all of their council Tax paid. However even if a person does not get this part of the pension credit, council tax may still be reduced or paid for. To find out a person should contact their local council and ask for information about this benefit. The details will be on a person's council tax bill.

Third Floor benefits.

This refers to benefits that are not means tested. In others words they do not take into consideration a person's income or their savings. This includes benefits such as:

The Attendance Allowance. This is payable to people with a disability, such as dementia, over the age of 65 who need support to look after themselves. This benefit is paid at various levels. This depends on a person's care needs. People with dementia living in a care home can still claim this benefit if they are self funding.

The Disability Living Allowance. This allowance is applicable to younger people with dementia i.e. below the age of 65. As well as care needs this benefit consider a persons' mobility. For example, for people with dementia who cannot walk or have difficulty in walking. Both of these benefits are paid at different rates depending on a person's needs.

Third Floor benefits can be received as well as floor one and two benefits. However a person does not need to claim from the other floors to get to level three benefits.

Potentially a person could receive benefits from all three floors such as the State Retirement Pension, Pension Credit and Attendance Allowance.

Advice

Advice about finances can be sought from a wide range of services including the Department of Work and pensions, which includes the Jobcentre Plus network for younger people with dementia and the Pensions service for older people, professional advisors, legal professionals and charitable organisations. For example the Alzheimer's Society provides a free range of leaflets explaining benefits.

These are just some possible contacts regarding advice about benefits.

Benefits Enquiry Lines.
These free phone services provide information about benefits, It also useful because advice can be given about the completion of forms over the telephone.

Phone: 0800 882200

Disability Living Allowance and Attendance Allowance Help line.
0845 712 3456

Carers Allowance
01253 856123

The Pension Service
0845 606 0265

Citizen's Advice Bureau.

Advisers can give provide free information about accessing services and benefits

Care Aware

Provides independent advice on funding of long term care, benefit entitlements and legal issues.

Senior Line 0808 800 6565 0076

Citizen's Advice Bureau.

Look in local telephone directories or on website for local bureau's

www.nacab.org.uk

Care Aware

Phone: 0875 134925. Calls charged at national rate.

Paying for a Care Home

For many people, moving into a care home can be a very difficult time. Before this is done it is worth considering the other options available such as sheltered housing, domiciliary care or respite care.

However if it is felt that moving into a care home is the right choice then it is worth contacting the local council social service department and asking for an assessment of needs. Usually an individual from the social services department should visit the person to find out what help is required. It is possible that a person may receive assistance with the costs of a care home if the council assesses this is a need. How much support received will depend on a person's income and savings. Usually if a person has savings of above £25,000 they will have to pay the full fees of a care home. If a person owns their home then this will often count as capital unless a person's partner or close relative over 60 or under 16 lives in the house.

If a person has savings below £8,000 then this should not be taken into consideration by the council. However a person weekly income will be taken into considerations, including any benefits.

A person may be assessed as having nursing care needs. If this is the case a person may need to move into a nursing home, and it is possible that some funding will come from the NHS.

Whoever pays for the care home it is important that the person with dementia has the opportunity to choose the home suitable for them.

The Elderly Accommodation Counsel has a list of care homes in the UK. (Telephone 020 7820 1343 or www.housingcare.org)

Legislation

Mental Capacity Act 2005 aims to help people with dementia who have difficulty in making decisions. The act calls this 'lacking capacity'. Decisions can be made by services based on assumptions about a person based on their dementia, their age or behaviour rather then considering the whole person.

This act stresses that it is important to give people with dementia as much support as possible to make decisions. Also the act claims that when decisions are made for the person it must be in their 'best interests' and does not limit their freedom and rights.

The act has also created a number of new roles and responsibilities including:

The lasting power of attorney.
This is a legal document that allows a person with dementia to state who they want to make decisions for them when they no longer have the ability to do so. The decisions can be about financial arrangements, health, i.e. should a person receive an operation if they need to and welfare, such as deciding which is the best care home for the person to go to?

Independent Mental Capacity Advocate. This role involves an individual supporting someone with dementia who has no family or friends. They will help make decisions around issues that involve health and social care services such as moving into a care home or going into hospital.

The Mental Capacity Act

Advance decisions.
This regards decisions a person can make while they still have the capacity to do so.

Court of Protection.
This is a court that deals with issues surrounding the Mental Capacity Act.

The Mental Health Act 1983

This legislation makes it possible for a person with dementia to be detained in a mental health ward/ hospital where they will receive treatment, such as anti-psychotic medication. A person with dementia will only be detained if it is felt that the person is at serious risk from hurting themselves or other people.

There are a number of areas, or sections, in this act. We shall look at 2 and 3. Section 2 states that any application made for detainment needs to be considered by two doctors. The person with dementia can then be kept in hospital for a period of 28 days. The person's consent usually needs to be sought before treatment is given. Section 3 differs to section two because a person can be detained for a minimum of 6 months. Furthermore the person does not need to give consent for their treatment.

In 2008 a number of changes have been made to the act including:

- A new single definition of 'Mental Disorder". Before there were four.
- New Safeguards to try and protect the person.
- New roles that replace approved social workers and medical officers.

The Enduring Power of Attorney Act 1985 enables the position of an Enduring Power of Attorney to be created. This is an individual who can make decisions regarding a person with dementia's financial affairs – such as selling a person's property or looking after their bank account.

The Disability Discrimination Act 1995 was introduced to try and prevent discrimination based on a person's disability. This piece of legislations should protect people with dementia against discrimination in a number of ways. For example being refused accommodation at a hotel because the proprietor believes that a person could cause a 'disturbance' or not being allowed in a Taxi because the driver thinks the person with dementia might 'jump out'.

Human Rights Act 1998 stresses that everyone, including people with dementia, have certain human rights. Some of these rights include:

- The right of respect for private and family life.
- Freedom of thought, conscience and religion.
- Freedom of Expression.
- The right of people to freedom from torture and from inhuman or degrading treatment
- The prohibition of discrimination

However a decision was made by the House of Lords in June 2007 that people with dementia who lived in private care homes were not covered by the Human Rights Act. The Lords claimed that the Act only covers public organisations such as council owned care homes, and not privately run services. This means that people who are evicted from private run care homes can not have their eviction overruled on the grounds that it breaking their human rights.

Care Standards Act (2000) developed a framework that care services care could follow. This framework includes a number of standards that services needed to achieve known as The National Minimum Standards. Regulatory bodies, such as CSCI, use these standards as a way of evaluating the support and care being given. This means that different providers are all judged by the same national standards.

The final chapter looks at the future of dementia care.

Chapter Ten

The Future

This final chapter examines what the future of dementia care in the UK could possibly hold.

Obviously nobody can predict the future but it seems certain that the number of people with dementia will significantly grow over the next twenty years as the aging population increases. However it appears that the future may be a mixture of progression and set backs.

Every cloud......

Many of the people who now have dementia have already been through a war that they were lucky to survive. Now 60 years later people with dementia, their families, carers and many professionals are faced with yet another war to fight. This time though, it involves fighting for their rights and quality care in the UK. At the moment the outcome has still not yet been decided. There are many obstacles still to be achieved including:

The need for quality Health and Social Care.

The current situation, regarding services for people with dementia and their families, certainly could be improved. A number of reports detailed overleaf have recognised the need for improved services for older people with dementia.

(The Audit Commission's 2002 *Forget Me Not report*, the National Service Frameworks on mental health, older people and long-term conditions and *"A new ambition for old age"* 2006). A report published by the National Audit Office in 2007, *"Improving services and support for people with dementia"* has suggested that only 25-50% of people with dementia ever receive a diagnosis. In the UK it takes much longer for a diagnosis to be given and there are less people who receive the anti dementia drugs compared to a number of other European countries

"It's an outrage….my Dad has worked all his life. Now when he needs something back he can't get it"

"I know not everyone benefits from these drugs. One of my residents had quite nasty side effects when she was taking it"

The right to the anti- dementia drugs on an NHS prescription.
In chapter 6 it was discussed how the National Institute for Clinical Excellence has advised that the anti-dementia drugs are not prescribed on the NHS for people in the early or late stages of dementia. The Alzheimer's Society, with others, challenged the advice given by NICE at the High Court..

However in August 2007 a ruling by the High Court upheld NICE's decision. Despite this Doctors can still prescribe the medication if they feel it is right for their patient

The right to be covered by the Human Rights Act. The House of Lords ruled in 2007 that people with dementia living in privately owned care homes did not have protection under the Human Rights Act. (See previous chapter)

The right to be treated as an individual. In 2007 the MP, Macolm Wicks, claimed that people with dementia should be electronically tagged so that their movements can be tracked. This would involve using the same equipment as used on young offenders. Although this may benefit some people with dementia, the question has to be asked if it would help all?

........has a silver Lining.

Despite many battles still needing to be won progress has started. For example In August, 2007 the Government announced that it was going to undertake the first national dementia strategy. This project aims to:

- Improve public and professional awareness about the reality of dementia.
- Concentrate on improving early diagnosis.
- Emphasise and encourage health & social care cooperation of services for people with dementia and their carers.

The project will be undertaken with the Care Services Improvement Partnership (CSIP) and a number of other organisations, such as Age concern and the Alzheimer's Society, to try and deliver improvements in dementia care, both nationally and locally. (CSIP is an organisation that was developed in 2005 to help improve care services).

This is a step forward because it shows that the Government is starting to recognise the massive impact dementia will have on us all over the coming years.

Furthermore political pressure is growing on the Government to increase the amount of funding into dementia. MPs, including the Shadow Health Secretary, have called for the need for more investment into research.

Currently the amount of money being spent in the UK into Alzheimer's is signfanctly less compared to cancer care

Nevertheless other countries, such as the US and Australia, are producing potentially promising findings. These include looking into:

- **A possible vaccination**. A study undertaken in the US found that an antibody stopped the harmful tau protein from developing inside the brain cells of mice.

- **Screening** for Alzheimer's is also being researched into in the US. This has included looking at skin cells and undertaking blood tests.

- **New drug treatments** are being explored. For example in Australia scientists have suggested that chemicals, found in athlete's foot treatments, may eventually be developed into a drug for people with dementia. Also new research gives hope that a new drug, called Rember, could help slow the progression of Alzheimer's, by tackling the protein tangles that cause brain cell death

It is clear that there are lots of avenues being explored in finding treatments or possible preventions. However it is important to realise that a lot of these studies are still in the very early stages and more research needs to be done before these treatments and preventions are safe for people with dementia.

Changing views.

With the emergence of person-centred care (Chapter five) many people's perception about people with dementia has changed. More services are now focusing on the person and their needs rather then the restricted ideas of the past.

Dementia and Alzheimer's is being featured more heavily in the media. More people with dementia are openly talking about their experiences. All of this can only help in changing people's views about dementia from something that should be feared to something that needs to be understood.

The future of dementia care remains uncertain but as one family member said:

"I can't give up on him…I have to carry on or else what is the point".

Index

Emerald Publishing
www.emeraldpublishing.co.uk

106 Ladysmith Road
Brighton BN2 4EG

Other titles in the Emerald Series:

Law

Guide to Bankruptcy
Conducting Your Own Court case
Guide to Consumer law
Creating a Will
Guide to Family Law
Guide to Employment Law
Guide to European Union Law
Guide to Health and Safety Law
Guide to Criminal Law
Guide to Landlord and Tenant Law
Guide to the English Legal System
Guide to Housing Law
Guide to Marriage and Divorce
Guide to The Civil Partnerships Act
Guide to The Law of Contract
The Path to Justice
You and Your Legal Rights

Health

Guide to Combating Child Obesity
Asthma Begins at Home

Music
How to Survive and Succeed in the Music Industry

General
A Practical Guide to Obtaining probate
A Practical Guide to Residential Conveyancing
Writing The Perfect CV
Keeping Books and Accounts-A Small Business Guide
Business Start Up-A Guide for New Business
Finding Asperger Syndrome in the Family-A Book of Answers

For details of the above titles published by Emerald go to:

www.emeraldpublishing.co.uk